The Ultimate Mediterranean Dash Diet Recipe Book

Boost Your Metabolism and Enjoy Your Meals with Incredibly Tasty Mediterranean Dash Diet Dishes

Kathyrn Solano

Table of contents

Great Mediterranean Diet Recipes

Pomegranate Avocado Salsa

Preparation time: 10 minutes

Cooking time: 10 minutes

Servings: 6

Ingredients:

1/3 cup red onion diced

1/3 cup chopped cilantro

Two pomegranates sliced

One jalapeno chopped

One avocado

Juice of 1 lime

1 tsp sea salt

Directions: Mix all the ingredients and serve.

Nutrition Info: Calories: 136 kcal Fat: 6 g Protein: 2 g Carbs: 21 g Fiber: 6 g

White Bean Bruschetta

Preparation time: 5 minutes

Cooking time: 10minutes

Servings: 6

Ingredients:

1 -2 clove garlic sliced

1 cup cannellini beans, cooked

½ tsp red pepper flakes

2 tbsp balsamic vinegar

2 tbsp olive oil

2 tbsp basil leaves

6 slices Italian bread

garlic

Salt to taste

Pepper to taste

Directions: Mix all the items in a jar except bread. Toast the bread and spread the mixture, and serve.

Nutrition Info: Calories: 137 kcal Fat: 5.5 g Protein: 4.1 g Carbs: 17.3 g Fiber: 2.8 g

Baked Fish Fillets

Preparation time: 10 minutes

Cooking time: 20 minutes

Servings: 6

Ingredients:

2 tbsp lemon juice

2 lb mackerel fillets

1 tsp salt

1 tbsp vegetable oil

¼ cup butter, melted

⅛ tsp paprika

⅛ tsp black pepper

Directions: Mix all the items in a bowl except fillets. Coat fillets with the mixture and bake in a preheated oven at 350 degrees for 25 minutes.

Nutrition Info: Calories: 399 kcal Fat: 31 g Protein: 28.8 g Carbs: 0.5 g Fiber: 0 g

Black Bean-Salmon Stir-Fry

Preparation time: 5 minutes

Cooking time: 20 minutes

Servings: 4

Ingredients:

2 tsp cornstarch

2 tbsp rice vinegar

2 tbsp sauce black bean garlic

12 oz mung bean sprouts

1 tbsp canola oil

1 tbsp rice wine

1 lb salmon

One pinch of red pepper

1 cup diced scallions

¼ cup of water

Directions:

Mix all the ingredients except salmon and set aside. The sauce is ready.

Cook salmon in heated oil for three minutes from each side.

Add the sauce to salmon and cook for a minute.

Mix in scallions and beans and cook for five minutes.

Nutrition Info: Calories: 330 kcal Fat: 19.4 g Protein: 26.7 g Carbs: 11.8 g Fiber: 2.7 g

Michael Symon's Grilled Salmon and Zucchini Salad

Preparation time: 8 minutes

Cooking time: 8 minutes

Servings: 4

Ingredients:

¼ cup chopped fresh dill

¼ cup sliced almonds, toasted

½ tsp black pepper, divided

¾ tsp kosher salt, divided

One lemon

3 cups sliced zucchini

3 tbsp olive oil, divided

24 oz salmon fillets

Directions:

Coat fillets with salt, pepper, and oil and grill over a preheated grill for five minutes for each side. Transfer in a plate.

Mix all the remaining ingredients and pour over fillets.

Nutrition Info: Calories: 379 kcal Fat: 22.7 g Protein: 38.2 g Carbs: 4.8 g Fiber: 1.6 g

Grilled Salmon with Mustard & Herbs

Preparation time: 5 minutes

Cooking time: 40 minutes

Servings: 4

Ingredients:

¼ tsp salt

One clove garlic

1 lb salmon

1 tbsp Dijon mustard

Two lemons sliced

30 sprigs mixed herbs

Directions:

Arrange a layer of lemon followed by herbs on a baking tray.

Mix garlic with salt and coat over salmon.

Place the salmon on herbs.

Place the pan in the grill and cook for 25 minutes.

Nutrition Info: Calories: 138 kcal Fat: 4.2 g Protein: 22.7 g Carbs: 1.1 g Fiber: 0.1 g

Japanese Salmon & Soba Noodle Salad

Preparation time: 10 minutes

Cooking time: 10 minutes

Servings: 4

Ingredients:

1 1/2 tbsp rice vinegar

1 tsp soy sauce

2 tbsp canola oil

2 tsp sesame oil

200 g snow peas sliced

250 g soba noodles

Three salmon fillets

Four green onions sliced

60 g baby spinach leaves

Directions: Bake the fillets wrapped in foil in a preheated oven at 180 degrees for five minutes.

Cook peas in boiling water for two minutes and drain them.

Now cook noodles in the same water for five minutes.

Now mix everything in a bowl and serve.

Nutrition Info: Calories: 958 kcal Fat: 27 g Protein: 38 g Carbs: 2 g Fiber: 5 g

Lemony Lentil Salad with Salmon

Preparation time: 5 minutes

Cooking time: 30 minutes

Servings: 6

Ingredients:

2 tsp Dijon mustard

14 oz salmon

30 oz lentils, rinsed

One diced red bell pepper

One pepper to taste

1 cup diced seedless cucumber

½ cup chopped red onion

1/3 cup lemon juice

1/3 cup olive oil

1/3 cup chopped dill

¼ tsp salt

Directions: Mix all the items in a bowl and serve.

Nutrition Info: Calories: 355 kcal Fat: 18.1 g Protein: 24 g Carbs: 24.4 g Fiber: 8.6 g

Oven-Poached Salmon Fillets

Preparation time: 5 minutes

Cooking time: 30 minutes

Servings: 4

Ingredients:

2 tbsp pepper

2 tbsp dry white wine

1 lb salmon fillet

1 Lemon wedges, for garnish

1 2 tbsp chopped shallot

¼ tsp salt

Directions: Whisk all the items except salmon in a bowl.
Put salmon in baking tray sprayed with oil with skin placed
downwards.
Pour the bowl content over the salmon and bake for 25 minutes
in a preheated oven at 425 degrees.
Serve with wedges.

Nutrition Info: Calories: 246 kcal Fat: 15.2 g Protein: 23.3 g
Carbs: 1.1 g Fiber: 0.1 g

Salmon and Cucumber Salad

Preparation time: 8 minutes

Cooking time: 35 minutes

Servings: 4

Ingredients:

Sauce

1/4 tsp kosher salt

2 tsp lemon juice

13 tsp pepper

1 tbsp olive oil

1 tbsp chopped dill

1 cup yogurt

 Cucumber salad

2 tsp olive oil

2 tsp chopped flat-leaf parsley

2 tsp chopped chives

13 tsp pepper

13 tsp kosher salt

1.5 tsp minced shallot

¾ tsp lemon juice

½ lb English cucumbers

Salmon and serving

¼ tsp kosher salt

¼ tsp pepper

1 tbsp olive oil

Four salmon fillets

Dill sprigs

Directions: Mix all the ingredients of the sauce list in a bowl. The sauce is ready.

Combine all the items of salad in a bowl and set aside. The salad and dressing are ready.

Place fish with skin placed downwards on a baking tray.

Grill the fillets for 15 minutes.

Place the grilled fillets on a plate and drizzle salad and dressing over it; serve.

Nutrition Info: Calories: 380 kcal Fat: 4.8 g Protein: 34 g Carbs: 5.6 g Fiber: 0.4 g

Salmon, Lentil & Pomegranate Salad

Preparation time: 15 minutes

Cooking time: 0 minute

Servings: 2

Ingredients:

One garlic clove chopped

One red onion sliced

1 tsp clear honey

One pomegranate

140 g hot-smoked salmon

2 tbsp olive oil

2 tbsp chopped tarragon

20 g flat-leaf parsley

400 g lentil

juice ½ lemon

toasted pitta bread, to serve

Directions:

Combine all the ingredients in a bowl and toss well.

Serve and enjoy it.

Nutrition Info: Calories: 382 kcal Fat: 18 g Protein: 27 g
Carbs: 14 g Fiber: 11 g

Salmon and pumpkin salad with chili jam

Preparation time: 30 minutes

Cooking time: 30 minutes

Servings: 2

Ingredients:

lime

coriander (chopped to serve)

700 g pumpkin

Four salmon fillets

200 g green beans

125 g baby spinach

1 tbsp olive oil

One sliced Spanish onion

Dressing

2 tbsp lime juice

1/2 cup vegetable stock (liquid)

1 tbsp fish sauce

1 tbsp chili jam

1 tbsp brown sugar

Directions:

Combine all the items of dressing in a pan and boil it for few minutes. The dressing is ready.

Drizzle oil over pumpkin and roast in a preheated oven at 200 degrees for 25 minutes.

Add peas to boiling water and cook for five minutes.

Cook salmon in a heated pan for five minutes.

Now mix all the items in a bowl and pour dressing.

Nutrition Info: Calories: 477 kcal Fat: 28 g Protein: 31 g Carbs: 28 g Fiber: 5 g

Salmon with Pomegranate Molasses Glaze

Preparation time: 5 minutes

Cooking time: 15 minutes

Servings: 3

Ingredients:

1/2 tsp salt

1/4 cup pomegranate molasses

1/4 tsp cornstarch

2 tsp brown sugar

Four boneless salmon fillets

Black pepper

pomegranate seeds for garnish

Mint for garnishing

Directions:

Whisk pepper, sugar, salt, and starch in a bowl. Coat fillets with the mixture.

Fry the fillets in heated oil for five minutes.

Transfer the fillets to the baking tray. Drizzle pomegranate molasses over fillets.

Bake in a preheated oven at 400 degrees for 15 minutes.

Nutrition Info: Calories: 301 kcal Fat: 10 g Protein: 33 g Carbs: 15 g Fiber: 1 g

Scallops and Summer Vegetable Skillet

Preparation time: 15 minutes

Cooking time: 15 minutes

Servings: Adjustable

Ingredients:

1 1/2 cup diced zucchini

1 cup corn kernels

One sliced cherry tomatoes

1 lb scallops

1 tbsp olive oil

Three cloves garlic minced

3 tbsp diced shallots

3 tbsp salted butter

Salt to taste

pepper to taste

Directions: Cook scallops in a heated oven over medium flame for three minutes. Transfer it to a plate. Sauté shallots and garlic in the same pan over medium flame. Stir in zucchini and tomatoes for ten minutes. Mix in corn, salt, and black pepper. Add scallop and cook for five minutes.

Nutrition Info: Calories: 550 kcal Fat: 26 g Protein: 41 g Carbs: 41 g Fiber: 4 g

Tuna Patties

Preparation time: 15 minutes

Cooking time: 10 minutes

Servings: 4

Ingredients:

3 tbsp vegetable oil

3 tbsp grated Parmesan cheese

3 tbsp diced Onion

15 oz tuna

2 tsp lemon juice

Two eggs

10 tbsp bread crumbs

One pinch of black pepper

Directions: Whisk all the items in a bowl.

Make patties out of the mixture.

Fry the patties in heated oil over medium flame for five minutes.

Nutrition Info: Calories: 324 kcal Fat: 1.5 g Protein: 31.3 g Carbs: 13 g Fiber: 0.83 g

Whole Salmon Fillet with Crispy Lemon & Basil Crumb Topping

Preparation time: 15 minutes

Cooking time: 18 minutes

Servings: 4

Ingredients:

Salt to taste

black pepper to taste

Two cloves garlic

1.45 lb salmon fillet

1 tbsp lemon juice

1 tbsp lemon thyme

1 lb asparagus

One lemon, zested

1 cup bread crumbs

½ tsp salt

½ tsp black pepper

1/3 cup grated Parmesan cheese

1/3 cup chopped fresh basil

¼ cup olive oil, divided

Directions:

Season salmon with oil, pepper, and salt.

Shift the salmon in the pan.

Mix asparagus with oil and salt and place around salmon.

Blend garlic, cheese, basil, thyme, lemon juice, zest, salt, and pepper in a food processor.

Pour the mixture over salmon.

Bake in the oven for 20 minutes.

Nutrition Info: Calories: 449 kcal Fat: 30.5 g Protein: 32.3 g Carbs: 11.7 g Fiber: 2.9 g

Seafood paella

Preparation time: 15 minutes

Cooking time: 55 minutes

Servings: 6

Ingredients:

Saffron Broth

Two ¼ cups chicken broth

2 tsp olive oil

1 lb jumbo shrimp

½ teaspoon saffron threads

Paella

salt to taste

8 oz sliced chorizo sausage

Two cloves garlic, minced

1 1/3 cups Arborio rice

1 tsp paprika

1 tbsp olive oil

One sliced red bell pepper

One pinch of cayenne pepper

½ yellow onion, diced

½ cup green peas

Directions:

Fry chorizo in heated oil for three minutes.

Mix in onions and cook for three more minutes.

Stir in rice and peas and toss well.

Place shrimp over rice and bake for twenty minutes.

Nutrition Info: Calories: 476 kcal Fat: 19.3 g Protein: 26.3 g Carbs: 47 g Fiber: 2 g

Thyme-Scented Salmon with White Bean Salad

Preparation time: 15 minutes

Cooking time: 0 minute

Servings: 4

Ingredients:

Bean Salad

3 tbsp lemon juice

2 tsp chopped parsley

2 tsp chopped mint

2 tsp chopped basil

2 tbsp water

Two garlic cloves, minced

1 tbsp olive oil

15 oz cannellini beans

½ cup chopped shallots

½ cup chopped carrot

1/3 cup chopped celery

Salmon

Four salmon fillets

3 tbsp lemon juice

2 tsp chopped thyme

13 tsp black pepper

1 tsp chopped parsley

½ tsp salt

Directions:

Cook celery, carrot, shallots, and garlic in heated oil over medium flame for five minutes. Mix all the ingredients and cook. Place the mixture in salmon. Bake salmon in a preheated oven at 375 degrees for 15 minutes.

Nutrition Info: Calories: 414 kcal Fat: 17 g Protein: 41 g Carbs: 22 g Fiber: 5 g

Curry Chicken Salad

Preparation time: 15 minutes

Cooking time: 15 minutes

Servings: 6

Ingredients:

Three cooked chicken breasts

2/3 cup chopped celery

2 tbsp lemon juice

1/4 tsp black pepper

1/4 cup sliced chives

1/3 cup raisins

1/2 tsp salt

1/2 cup roasted salted cashews

1/2 cup mayonnaise

1 tbsp yellow curry powder

One tart apple

Directions: Whisk all the items in the bowl and serve.

Nutrition Info: Calories: 540 kcal Fat: 5 g Protein: 65 g Carbs: 11 g Fiber: 1 g

Grilled Indian Chicken

Preparation time: 35 minutes

Cooking time: 10 minutes

Servings: 4

Ingredients:

• 4 boneless chicken breasts

Marinade

1/4 tsp cayenne pepper

1/2 tsp ginger

1/2 cup plain yogurt

1 tsp cumin

1 tsp coriander

1 tbsp paprika

1 tbsp onion powder

1 tbsp minced garlic

1 tbsp lemon juice

1 tbsp garam masala

1 tbsp cilantro leaves

Directions: Combine all the items in a bowl and set aside. Grill chicken over a grill for seven minutes from both sides.

Nutrition Info: Calories: 279 kcal Fat: 20 g Protein: 20 g Carbs: 6 g Fiber: 2 g

Hearty Turkey Stew

Preparation time: 10 minutes

Cooking time: 60 minutes

Servings: 4

Ingredients:

100 g sliced bacon lardons

1/3 cup heavy cream

1 tbsp butter

One leek

Two sliced carrots

Two stalks celery diced

Two cloves garlic pressed

2 tbsp flour, heaped

4 cups chicken or turkey stock

2 cups cooked turkey

Two chopped potatoes

Two bay leaves

1 tbsp thyme leaves

1 tbsp chopped parsley

salt to taste

pepper to taste

Directions:

Fry bacon in butter over medium flame. Stir in leeks, carrots, thyme, and celery, and cook for five minutes. Mix garlic and cook again for one minute. Add flour, pepper, and salt.

Mix potatoes, bay leaves, and turkey and cook for 50 minutes. Add heavy cream and serve.

Nutrition Info: Calories: 278 kcal Fat: 22 g Protein: 22 g Carbs: 25 g Fiber: 5 g

Herb and Orange Chicken

Preparation time: 10 minutes

Cooking time: 60 minutes

Servings: 4

Ingredients:

1/4 cup ghee

3 1/2 oranges

4.5 lb chicken

Three yellow potatoes

Two stems of rosemary

Six stems of thyme

salt & pepper

Directions:

Heat orange juice in ghee over medium flame and set aside.

Place chicken, potatoes, orange slices, thyme, and rosemary.

Bake for one hour and serve with orange sauce.

Nutrition Info: Calories: 705 kcal Fat: 53 g Protein: 46 g Carbs: 8.8 g Fiber: 2.5 g

Pomegranate Walnut & Chicken Stew

Preparation time: 15 minutes

Cooking time: 75 minutes

Servings: 5

Ingredients:

2 cups California walnuts

pinch salt

pepper

2 tbsp olive oil

1 tbsp butter

Four cloves garlic chopped

1 tsp turmeric

1 tsp cumin

One cinnamon stick

½ tsp nutmeg

½ tsp black pepper

orange zest

2 cups chicken stock

2 tbsp maple

1 ½ tsp salt

One chickpea

serve with Persian Rice

Garnish using chopped Italian parsley

Garnish with pomegranate seeds

1–1 ½ lb chicken thighs

3 cups yellow onion, diced

1/4 cup pomegranate molasses

Directions:

Roast the walnuts over medium flame.

Blend the roasted walnuts.

Cook chicken in a Dutch oven in heated oil. Set aside.

Fry onions in heated oil for five minutes.

Stir in garlic and sauté for five minutes.

Mix cinnamon, nutmeg, cumin, zest, and turmeric and sauté for a minute.

Pour in stock, chicken, syrup, molasses, walnuts, salt, and simmer for 45 minutes.

Add the chickpeas and boil it for 15 minutes.

Nutrition Info: Calories: 532 kcal Fat: 37 g Protein: 23.2 g Carbs: 29.8 g Fiber: 5.7 g

Roasted Chicken and White Bean Medley

Preparation time: 20 minutes

Cooking time: 60 minutes

Servings: 4

Ingredients:

Eight teaspoons Dijon mustard

Eight skin-on bone-in chicken thighs (about 2 pounds)

Two tablespoons olive oil

Two tablespoons coarsely chopped fresh parsley

Two tablespoons capers with brine

2 (15-ounce) cans white beans, drained and rinsed

1/2 teaspoon freshly ground black pepper

One large lemon, thinly sliced, seeds removed

1 1/2 teaspoons kosher salt

Directions:

Preheat oven to 425 °F.

In a baking dish, toss capers, beans & distribute them on the tray.

Spread mustard in beans & capers on the skin of every chicken.

Put lemon pieces all around & beneath chicken & add insufficient water.

Spice the dish with black pepper & sea salt & spray chicken with oil.

Insert the instant-read thermometer in chicken and roast it until skin becomes brown for thirty-five minutes

Switch the pan on the lower rack of the oven if the chicken starts to smoke while finishing the frying process.

Place prepared chicken in a bowl and decorate it with slices of lemon, capers, & beans. Put chicken sauce across the bowl and sprinkle it with parsley.

Nutrition Info: Calories: 302 kcal Fat: 7 g Protein: 26 g Carbs: 34 g Fiber: 7.7 g

South-Western Chicken Salad

Preparation time: 10 minutes

Cooking time: 0 minutes

Servings: 6

Ingredients:

1 cup crushed tortilla chips

1 and 1/2 cups black beans

1 and 1/2 cups corn

One avocado, diced

One teaspoon minced garlic

1/2 cup plain Greek yogurt (use nonfat)

1/2 jalapeño, finely diced

1/2 red onion, diced

Two teaspoons apple cider vinegar

Two heaping teaspoons taco seasoning (use mild)

Two teaspoons honey

Two tomatoes, diced

3 Tablespoons extra virgin olive oil

3/4 cup shredded cheddar cheese

6 cups chopped romaine lettuce

6 cups cubed cooked chicken*

Dressing

handful chopped cilantro

juice of 1 lime

salt, to taste and if needed

Directions:

Add all the ingredients to the bowl and mix them except salt

Pour the dressing over the salad and toss it.

Serve it cold.

Nutrition Info: Calories: 741 kcal Fat: 39 g Protein: 51 g Carbs: 51 g Fiber: 17.5 g

The best turkey chili ever

Preparation time: 15 minutes

Cooking time: 60 minutes

Servings: 1

Ingredients:

Three cloves of garlic, minced

Two teaspoons hot sauce

Two tablespoons olive oil

Two tablespoons chili powder

2 pounds lean ground turkey

2 cups chicken or vegetable broth

1/2 teaspoon cayenne pepper (optional)

One yellow pepper, chopped

One yellow bell pepper, chopped

One teaspoon garlic powder

One teaspoon dried oregano

One teaspoon dried basil

One tablespoon brown sugar

One sweet onion, finely chopped

One red bell pepper, chopped

1 1/2 teaspoon sea salt

28oz crushed tomatoes

28oz black beans, drained

15oz petite diced tomatoes

15oz of kidney or pinto beans

Toppings: Sour cream, green onions, limes, shredded cheddar cheese

Directions:

Heat the olive oil in a heavy bottom pot over medium-high & heat it till it shimmers.

Add-In the ground turkey & simmer for 9 minutes, smashing it individually with a wooden spoon's help until it turned brown.

Add more olive oil if needed & whisk in onions & garlic.

Cook for 3 minutes before soften & fragrant.

Add peppers & again cook for three more minutes.

Place the fried turkey in the pot again & then add the remaining ingredients to it.

Stir & bring to a boil once combined.

Simmer this till the chili cooked completely 7 left it uncovered for 45 to 65 minutes until it becomes dense

Nutrition Info: Calories: 481 kcal Fat: 23 g Protein: 45 g Carbs: 782 mg Fiber: 25 g

Warm Chicken Pasta Salad

Preparation time: 5 minutes

Cooking time: 18 minutes

Servings: 3

Ingredients:

375g dried rigatoni pasta

500g Lilydale Free Range Chicken Breast, trimmed

One medium brown onion, thinly sliced

One garlic clove, crushed

200g semi-dried tomatoes, drained, chopped

300ml pure cream

50g baby rocket

1/2 teaspoon dried chili flakes

1/4 cup olive oil

Directions:

Take frypan and cook pasta until it becomes soft to follow the pasta packet's instructions and drain the remaining water. Along with that, heat 1 tbsp. Oil in a pan and add chicken to it. Cook every side until it is completely cooked. Remove frypan from the stove, cover it & set it aside for 6 minutes.

Take the remaining oil in a frypan, heat it over medium heat, and then add the onion. Cook for 4 to 6 minutes, mix frequently, or till the onion has softened.

Onions, Garlic, & chili are added. Cook for 1 minute or till the smell is floral.

Now add cream, then cook for 4 to 6 minutes, or till the mixture thickens, stirring regularly.

Put a bowl of spaghetti, chicken, and rocket. Add the onions mixture. To combine, toss. Just serve.

Nutrition Info: Calories: 105 kcal Fat: 48 g Protein: 48 g Carbs: 85 g Fiber: 11 g

Glazed Venison Medallions

Preparation time: 5 minutes

Cooking time: 8 minutes

Servings: 2

Ingredients:

Freshly ground black pepper

2 tbsp red currant jelly

1 Tbsp olive oil

One pack of Silver Fern Farms Venison Medallions

½ cup reduced-salt chicken stock

Directions: Toss in olive oil & pepper with medallions. Place skillet on a high temperature. Fry it quickly on each side for 3-4 minutes.

Remove from frypan, cover, and leave for 3-4 minutes. Apply to the pan the red currant jelly & decreased-salt stock of chicken. Melt & Simmer till it is like a thick paste.

Sprinkle juices from pan with medallions and serve at your selection of seasonal vegetables or oven-baked potatoes.

Nutrition Info: Calories: 451 kcal Fat: 23 g Protein: 33 g Carbs: 63 g Fiber: 4.8 g

Venison Tenderloin

Preparation time: 20 minutes

Cooking time: 75 minutes

Servings: 6

Ingredients:

4 pounds venison tenderloin

2 sprigs fresh thyme

2 sprigs fresh rosemary

Two cloves garlic, crushed

Two bay leaves

One medium onion, chopped

1 cup red wine

½ cup apple cider vinegar

Directions:

Add red wine cider vinegar, garlic, bay leaves, thyme, rosemary & onion in a cup & blend them.

Move it to the large jar, & place in the bag the venison tenderloin.

Close it tightly, and make it airtight.

Then place the meat in a refrigerator for marination for at least 13 hours, turn it 2 or 3 times.

Preheated the oven to 325°F (165 °C).

Take Off meat away from the marinade & put it in a roasting rack.

Roast it for two to two and a half hours in the oven.

The Internal roasting temperature would be a minimum of 150 °F

Let the roast rest for 10 to 15 minutes before cutting.

Heat the sauce over low heat in a pan as the side roasts.

Boil till there is a 1/3 drop in the oil. Serve & Enjoy

Nutrition Info: Calories: 345 kcal Fat: 6.1 g Protein: 57 g Carbs: 3.4 g Fiber: 0.4 g

Seared venison with plum ginger sauce and vermicelli sauce

Preparation time: 10 minutes

Cooking time: 15 minutes

Servings: 2

Ingredients:

Vermicelli salad

One carrot grated

One red capsicum sliced

100 g snow peas sliced

100 g vermicelli noodles

Two tbsp Thai basil leaves chopped

Venison and plum sauce

¼ cup red wine

One clove garlic minced

One tablespoon soy sauce

One teaspoon ginger finely grated

Two tablespoons plum jam

300 g venison medallions

Dressing

½ teaspoon sesame oil

One tablespoon olive oil

One tablespoon soy sauce

One teaspoon plum jam

To serve

One tablespoon Thai basil leaves chopped
One tablespoon sesame seeds

Directions:
Bring to the boil a full pot.

Use a Proof heat Bowl, place the vermicelli noodles in the bowl and pour over the boiling water to cover them. Threads are detached by stirring, covering with a plate, and leaving until smooth, around 4 minutes. Threads are shortened by cutting the threads from different places using kitchen scissors. Apply oil in a small amount to avoid Sticking.

Use paper towels, Dry the venison, and season it with salt. Heat the saucepan to medium temperature. Toast sesame seeds until crispy and fragrant for 1 to 2 minutes. Add a drizzle of oil and raise the heat. Once cooked, grill the venison for 2 to 3 minutes on both sides. Cover the venison with foil.

Return the pan to low heat for the plum sauce and apply a small amount of oil. Fry the ginger and garlic for 30 seconds, stir-fry the red wine, and boil until halved. Now add plum jelly, fresh plums, and soy sauce and boil until slightly thickened, and stir for around 1 minute. Use black pepper for seasoning. If the sauce gets too thick and jam-like, give a splash of water to thin it out to a decent pouring consistency. Stir in the sleeping venison juices.

Mix all of the ingredients in a big dish. Add all the salad ingredients leftover, the noodles, and toss to coat. Season with salt and pepper.

Divide the vermicelli salad between the plates to serve. Cover with venison and drizzle all over the sauce with plum. Sprinkle the Thai basil and sesame seeds.

Nutrition Info: Calories: 495 kcal Fat: 18 g Protein: 36 g Carbs: 12 g Fiber: 1.1 g

Venison Stir-Fry

Preparation time: 20 minutes

Cooking time: 5 minutes

Servings: 4

Ingredients:

Marinade

1/2 teaspoon salt

Two tablespoons Shaoxing wine or dry sherry

Three tablespoons soy sauce

One tablespoon potato starch

Stir fry

1 1/2 cups peanut or other cooking oil

1 pound venison, trimmed of fat

1 to 4 fresh red chiles

One red or yellow bell pepper, sliced

Three garlic cloves, slivered

One bunch cilantro, roughly chopped

One tablespoon soy sauce

Two teaspoons sesame oil

Directions:

Cut the venison into small slivers between 1/4 inch or less and 1 to 3 inches in length from anywhere. Mix and set aside with the marinade as you cut out all the remaining ingredients.

Heat a big heavy pot with the peanut oil until it reaches 275 °F to 290 °F. Apply about 1/3 of venison to hot oil and use a chopstick or a butter knife to separate the meat slices. Let them sizzle for 30 - 60 seconds. Set aside and cook one-third at a time for the remaining venison.

Pour all but only three tablespoons of the oil out of it.

Keep the remaining oil hot. Add up the chiles and the bell peppers. Stir-fry for 90 seconds when it starts to burn, add garlic, and cook for an extra 30 seconds. Add the venison and fry for 90 seconds and stir.

Add the coriander and soy sauce and fry for the remaining 30 seconds before the coriander wilts. Turn the heat off, then whisk in the sesame oil. Serve with steamed rice at once.

Nutrition Info: Calories: 225 kcal Fat: 5 g Protein: 37 g Carbs: 6 g Fiber: 1 g

Lamb, apricot & shallot tagine

Preparation time: 30 minutes
Cooking time: 7 hrs. 30 minutes
Servings: 5-6

Ingredients:
1 tbsp clear honey
1 tbsp ras el hanout
One large leg of lamb, bone-in (about 2kg)
150ml hot chicken stock
Two preserved lemons
400g small apricot, halved and stoned
600g shallot, halved if particularly large
85g whole skinless almond
couscous and natural yogurt, to serve
little pack coriander leaves picked
For the marinade
1 tbsp ground cumin
2 tbsp clear honey
2 tsp coriander seed
2 tsp ground cinnamon
2 tsp ground ginger
4 tbsp olive oil
Four garlic cloves, crushed
pinch of saffron strands

Directions:

Cut the lamb's leg all over and put it in a large bag of food. Using the pestle and mortar, shatter the marinade ingredients simultaneously. Brush over the entire lamb with black pepper. Overnight, or up to 24 hours, to marinate.

Place the lamb in a large roasting tin, removing any residual marinade from the top. Use foil to protect the container, and close the foil from the ends. Cook for 6-7 hours, basting until the beef is extremely tender.

Drop the oven roasting tin and raise the oven to 200°C /180°C. Pour into a measuring jug the juices from the lamb, slightly cool it, and remove the fat off. Place the shallots with the lamb in the tin and toss in some of the juices to coat them. Roast the apricots and almonds for 15 mins, and then add them. Whisk the lemon, honey, ras el hanout, and stock in the cooking juices, then pour on the lamb and then roast again for 20 mins.

Leave it for 10 minutes, then scatter and eat with couscous and yogurt over the herbs.

Nutrition Info: Calories: 659 kcal Fat: 41 g Protein: 57 g Carbs: 18 g Fiber: 4 g

Flank Steak, Broccoli and Green Bean Stir-Fry

Preparation time: 15minutes

Cooking time: 12minutes

Servings:

Ingredients:

3 cups cooked brown rice

Two tablespoons vegetable oil

Two tablespoons rice vinegar

One ¼ pound lean beef flank steak

1 cup beef broth

One tablespoon cornstarch

One head broccoli, cut into florets (about 6 cups)

1 cup shredded carrot

½ teaspoon red pepper flakes

½ teaspoon Chinese five-spice powder

½ pound thin green beans, trimmed

½ large onion, sliced

½ cup sliced almonds

¼ teaspoon salt

¼ cup reduced-sodium soy sauce

Directions:

Combine the soy sauce, broth, 5-spice powder, vinegar, cornstarch, & the red chili flakes in a cup and place it aside.

Take a non-stick fry pan, add 1 tbsp of oil to it, and heat it.

Pepper the salted stir-fry flank steak & for 4 minutes. Remove to a tray.

Add the remaining one tbsp. Of oil in it, and then add broccoli, cabbage, green beans, & carrot. Stir-cook for 9 minutes or till it becomes soft & crisp.

Add ¼ cup of water at the last two minutes of cooking time. Now add a mixture of soya sauce& broth in it and then boil & simmer it for 2 minutes, until well dense. Stir in some stored juices & beef & heat up.

Decorate with the almonds & serve with the cooked brown rice instantly.

Nutrition Info: Calories: 388 kcal Fat: 15 g Protein: 29 g Carbs: 35 g Fiber: 6 g

Moroccan beef tagine

Preparation time: 25 minutes

Cooking time: 7 hrs

Servings: 4

Ingredients:

Marinade

pinch of sea salt

pinch of ground cardamon

1 tsp ground sweet paprika

1 tsp ground ginger

1 tsp ground cumin

1 tsp ground cinnamon

1 tsp dried rose petals

1 tbsp ras el hanout

1 tbsp olive oil

Tagine

One onion, peeled and chopped

1 tbsp olive oil for frying

400 g of chickpeas

400 g chopped tomatoes

150 g prunes, sliced

150 ml of beef stock

Two carrots sliced

Four small tomatoes quartered

400 g butternut squash, diced

600 g diced stewing beef

fresh coriander

Directions:

Combine all marinade items in a small glass. Take a dish, place beef in it, pour marinade all over it & mix it well for coating all-beef parts equally. Cover bowl with foil & refrigerate it for 3 to 4 hours. Take a frying pan, add oil in it, heat it, add onions and fry for 3 to 4 minutes, then add beef in it and fry it for 5 to 6 minutes until it turned brown. In a boiled slow oven dish, pass by the onion & beef. Add & stock the tinned tomatoes along with onions, quartered tomatoes &, stir well, add the onions, quartered tomatoes, & butternut squash, & then mix again. Turn on the auto mode, cover a slow cooker, & keep a dish simmer for 7 to 8 hours until the beef is very tender. Add the prunes & chickpeas for one hour till cooking ends.

Serve with splattered couscous with finely sliced coriander.

Nutrition Info: Calories: 565 kcal Fat: 15 g Protein: 56 g Carbs: 54 g Fiber: 2.1 g

Persian Roast Lamb

Preparation time: 20 minutes

Cooking time: 150 minutes

Servings: 8

Ingredients:

One large onion sliced or chopped

1 tbsp EV olive oil

1 tbsp ground cumin

1 tsp ground black pepper

1 tsp turmeric

One leg or shoulder of lamb

Two strips of fresh rosemary

2 Tbsp honey

2 Tbsp liquid saffron

250 ml of vegetable stock

4 tbsp pomegranate molasses

Five cloves garlic finely chopped or crushed

One lemon juice

Marinade

Directions:

Preheat micro to 180 deg C.

Make slashes.

Mix ingredients & rub them over the lamb.

Line sliced onions with a preferred dish.

Pour the stock.

Remember to Pour on onions.

Cover using foil & roast for 60 minutes.

Have the lamb wrapped in aluminum foil with a wonderful sauce.

Nutrition Info: Calories: 311 kcal Fat: 10 g Protein: 38 g Carbs: 15 g Fiber: 1 g

Stir-fried garlic chili beef and ong Choi

Preparation time: 8 minutes

Cooking time: 15 minutes

Servings: 2

Ingredients:

200g beef fillet, sliced into even-sized thin strips

Few pinches Chinese five-spice

Light soy sauce to season

1 tbsp groundnut oil

Four large garlic cloves, finely chopped

150 ong Choi, washed, leaves and stems cut across the stem in equal 10cm lengths (or use spinach or watercress)

One medium red chili, de-seeded and finely chopped

Toasted sesame oil, to season

Directions:

Season the beef with soy sauce. Toss well. Heat a saucepan. Add oil & garlic. Fry 30 sec. Add beef & stir. Apply one Choi & chili. Season with light soy sauce, sea salt, & sesame oil splashes for serving. Serve immediately & enjoy.

Nutrition Info: Calories: 270 kcal Fat: 17.7 g Protein: 24.6 g Carbs: 3.1 g Fiber: 0 g

Asian Broccoli and Ginger Salad

Preparation time: 10minutes

Cooking time: 10 minutes

Servings: 4

Ingredients:

Salt and pepper to taste

Three tablespoons low sodium soy sauce

Three tablespoons balsamic vinegar

Two cloves garlic minced

Two teaspoons brown sugar

2 cups sugar snap peas

1/4 cup almonds

One red pepper julienne cut

1 (12 ounces) bag broccoli coleslaw

One tablespoon fresh ginger

1 1/2 teaspoons sesame oil

Directions:

Mix soy sauce, garlic, sesame oil, vinegar, brown sugar, & ginger.

Put it aside for a while.

Steam sugar snaps for roughly 3-4 min.

For stopping the cooking process, immerse it in an ice bath.

Drain well.

Mix peas, almonds, broccoli coleslaw, red pepper & sesame ginger.

Dressing in a big dish.

Add salt to taste & black pepper powder.

Nutrition Info: Calories: 132 kcal Fat: 5.1 g Protein: 4.8 g Carbs: 17 g Fiber: 0 g

Avocado and three-bean salad

Preparation time: 15minutes
Cooking time: 15 minutes
Servings: 8

Ingredients:

salt and pepper to taste

juice of 2 limes

Two large avocados, peeled, pitted, and diced

Two cloves garlic, mashed or finely diced

12 grape or cherry tomatoes, halved

1/3 cup olive oil

One large orange or red bell pepper, diced

One bunch cilantro, chopped

15 oz kernel corn

15 oz red kidney beans

15 oz garbanzo beans

15 oz black beans

Directions:

Take a big bowl. Combine all ingredients. Refrigerate for 60 minutes before serving. Tossed it with lime. Serve & enjoy.

Nutrition Info: Calories: 258 kcal Fat: 18 g Protein: 10 g Carbs: 7 g Fiber: 13.6 g

Baked Adzuki Beans with Aubergine & Tomatoes

Preparation time: 8 minutes

Cooking time: 90 minutes

Servings: 6

Ingredients:

One bouquet garni (thyme, parsley, and bay leaf)

1 cup chicken stock (or one bouillon cube dissolved in 1 cup water)

1 cup dried adzuki beans

One onion, finely chopped

1/2 cup fresh grated parmesan cheese

1/2 teaspoon ground allspice

1/4 teaspoon red pepper flakes

Two cloves garlic, minced

Two sliced eggplants

2 1/2 cups canned chopped tomatoes

Four tablespoons fresh basil, shredded

Six tablespoons olive oil

kosher salt or sea salt

salt and pepper, to taste

Directions:

Add garlic & boil water. Reduce heat & simmer before beans become soft for 50 minutes. Preheat microwave to 375°. Heat olive oil in a frying pan on moderate heat. Move to bake dish. Heat leftover olive oil pan & sauté onion before it begins to soften. Add garlic & sauté for one min. Add tomatoes, red pepper flakes, salt, allspice, & black pepper. Blend well. Sprinkle with cheese & bake for 20 min. Serve & enjoy.

Nutrition Info: Calories: 344 kcal Fat: 17 g Protein: 13.5 g Carbs: 38 g Fiber: 11.7 g

Baked egg with cheddar and beef

Preparation time: 20 minutes

Cooking time: 20 minutes

Servings: 6

Ingredients:

Six eggs

1 lb beef

One chopped green pepper

Salt to taste

Pepper to taste

1 cup green beans

Cream of mushroom soup

1/2 cup shredded cheddar cheese

1 cup almond milk

1 tbsp vegetable oil

1 cup mushrooms

1 tsp onion powder

2 tbsp cornstarch

1/2 tsp salt

Directions:

Cook beef with beans and bell pepper. Crack eggs and cook for five minutes. Transfer the beef to the casserole and pour mushroom soup and toss. Bake in a preheated oven at 350 degrees for 20 minutes. Cream of Mushroom Soup Blend all the items of mushroom soup in the blender. Boil the mixture and simmer it for 12 minutes.

Nutrition Info: Calories: 610 kcal Fat:47 g Protein: 43 g Carbs: 5 g Fiber:0 g

Heavenly egg bake with pancakes

Preparation time: 15 minutes

Cooking time: 25 minutes

Servings: 8

Ingredients:

2 cups baking mix

2 cups shredded Cheddar cheese

1 cup milk

5 tbsp maple syrup

Two eggs

1.5 tbsp white sugar

12 slices cooked bacon

Directions:

Mix all the ingredients in a bowl and bake in a preheated oven at 350 degrees for 25 minutes.

Top with cheese and bacon and bake for five more minutes.

Nutrition Info: Calories: 311.1 kcal Fat: 15.8 g Protein: 11.7 g Carbs: 31.1 g Fiber: 0.5 g

Blueberry and vanilla scones

Preparation time: 15 minutes

Cooking time: 10 minutes

Servings: 8

Ingredients:

1/2 tsp baking powder

225 g Self-rising flour

One pinch of salt

2 tbsp soured cream

One egg

50 g caster sugar

75 g butter

75 g blueberries

1 tsp vanilla extract

Directions: Mix flour, salt, baking powder, sugar, butter, and blueberries in a bowl.

Whisk vanilla with cream and egg and add in flour mixture.

Make small rounded shapes and bake in a preheated oven at 200 degrees for 15 minutes.

Mix strawberries, sugar, and vanilla and make syrup.

Pour syrup over baked cookies and serve.

Nutrition Info: Calories: 267 kcal Fat: 2 g Protein: 5 g Carbs: 54 g Fiber: 1 g

Frittata with brie and bacon

Preparation time: 5 minutes

Cooking time: 20 minutes

Servings: 6

Ingredients:

1/2 tsp salt

1/2 tsp pepper

1/2 cup whipping cream

Eight slices bacon

Eight eggs

Two cloves garlic

4 oz brie

Directions:

Heat oil in a skillet over medium flame and saute bacon for five minutes. Transfer bacon to plate.

Mix egg, cream salt, bacon, pepper, and garlic and cook in heated oil over medium flame.

Broil bacon mixture for five minutes in broiler over a high flame.

Nutrition Info: Calories: 338 kcal Fat: 27 g Protein: 18 g Carbs: 1.8 g Fiber: 0.1 g

Coffee with butter

Preparation time: 5 minutes

Cooking time: 5 minutes

Servings: 1

Ingredients:

1 cup hot coffee

2 tbsp butter

1 tbsp coconut oil

Directions: Combine all the items in a blender and serve.

Nutrition Info: Calories: 230 kcal Fat: 25 g Protein: 0 g Carbs: 0 g Fiber: 0 g

Creamy Cheese Pancake

Preparation time: 2 minutes

Cooking time: 6 minutes

Servings: 4

Ingredients:

1 lb sea scallops

Four thyme

Salt to taste

Black pepper to taste

2 tbsp butter

Two lemons

1 tbsp olive oil

Directions:

Cook scallops for five minutes over a high flame in a skillet.

Stir in herbs and cook in butter for six minutes.

Squeeze lemon juice and serve.

Nutrition Info: Calories: 227 kcal Fat: 24.5 g Protein: 1.6 g Carbs:1.7 g Fiber: 6 g

Persimmon toast with cream

Preparation time: 5 minutes

Cooking time: 0 minutes

Servings: 1

Ingredients:

One sliced bread

1 Sour cream

1/2 Persimmon

1 Cinnamon

1 Granulated sugar

Directions:

Place cream over bread and lay persimmon slices.

Drizzle sugar and cinnamon.

Bake in preheated oven for five minutes at 250 degrees

Nutrition Info: Calories: 341 kcal Fat: 8 g Protein: 9 g Carbs: 58 g Fiber: 4 g

Tofu with mushrooms

Preparation time: 25 minutes

Cooking time: 17 minutes

Servings: 4

Ingredients:

pepper to taste

1 tbsp sweetener

1 tbsp Hoisin sauce

14 oz tofu

5 tbsp soy sauce

1 lb Cremini mushrooms

One pinch of red color

1 tbsp rice vinegar

2 tsp peanut oil

Three sliced ginger

1 tsp sesame oil

Three sliced garlic cloves

1/2 cup sliced green onions

Directions:

Marinate tofu with a mixture of vinegar, pepper, soy sauce, and sesame oil in a bowl.

Drain tofu after 30 minutes of marination.

Add agav to the marination mixture.

Sauté ginger and garlic in heated oil over medium flame.

Mix in tofu and cook for ten minutes.

After seven minutes, take out tofu and set aside.

Pour oil and add mushrooms and cook for five more minutes.

Again put tofu in the pan and cook.

Pour in sauce mixture and reduce the flame and cook for five minutes.

Stir in onions and cook for two minutes.

Serve and enjoy it.

Nutrition Info: Calories: 235 kcal Fat: 14 g Protein: 16 g Carbs: 11 g Fiber: 11 3 g

Ham spinach ballet

Preparation time: 10 minutes

Cooking time: 22 minutes

Servings: 6

Ingredients:

1/2 cup ham

1/4 tsp seasoned salt

1/2 tsp dry mustard

1.5 cups spinach

2 tbsp olive oil

Eight eggs

1/4 cup half and half

1/2 pound potatoes

Two green onions sliced

1/4 tsp black pepper

1/2 cup cheddar cheese divided

Directions:

Preheat the oven up to 400°F.

Heat olive oil in a skillet. Add potatoes & water. Season with salt & pepper

Now stir, Cover & cook (10-15 min) until softened.

Stir in ham, green & spinach along with onions until hot & spinach is wilted.

Take a bowl combine egg, dry mustard, & seasonings.

Pour on potato mixture & Top with the cheese.

Bake for 10-12 minutes until eggs are set.

Broil for 1-2 min.

Remove from oven & cool 5 min before cutting.

Serve warm and enjoy.

Nutrition Info: Calories: 191 kcal Fat: 13 g Protein: 11 g Carbs: 6 g Fiber: 1 g

Creamy parsley soutte

Preparation time: 5 minutes

Cooking time: 5 minutes

Servings: 4

Ingredients:

25 g flour

25 g butter

One handful parsley

salt to taste

1 cup milk

pepper (to taste)

Directions:

take saucepan & melt butter on moderate heat.

Stir in flour & mustard.

Stir thoroughly & form a thick paste.

Cook gently for 2-3 minutes.

Gradually whisk in milk.

Bring a boil, lower heat, & simmer 5 min,

The sauce should be quite & thick.

If too thick, then add a little more milk to have a smooth consistency.

Add parsley & stir well.

Season with a pinch of salt & black pepper grinds.

Taste & add more if needed.

Keep sauce warm.

Serve & enjoy.

Nutrition Info: Calories: 121 kcal Fat: 9 g Protein: 3 g Carbs: 8 g Fiber: 1 g

Quick McMuffins

Preparation time: 10 minutes

Cooking time: 15 minutes

Servings: 5

Ingredients:

Six slices of cheddar cheese

6 English Muffins

Six eggs

1 tbsp butter

6 Canadian Bacon

Directions:

Preheat the oven up to 400° F.

Arrange the Canadian Bacon on a wire rack, placed on a rimmed baking sheet.

Bake it until lightly browned 15 min.

Meanwhile, spray the muffin pan.

Break the egg into each cup of a muffin pan.

Add in the oven for 10 min for the bacon.

Split muffins into half.

Spread butter & arrange baking sheet.

Add to the bottom rack of the oven for 10 min.

Remove from oven & assemble Egg McMuffins.

Add a slice of cheesc.

Top with egg, followed by the slice.

Add another half of the English muffin on the top of the McMuffin.

Serve warm & enjoy.

Nutrition Info: Calories: 388 kcal Fat: 19 g Protein: 24 g Carbs: 27 g Fiber: 1 g

Egg fast snickerdoodle crepes

Preparation time: 5 minutes

Cooking time: 10 minutes

Servings: 4

Ingredients:

Crepes

1 tbsp sugar

butter

Six eggs

5 oz cream cheese

1 tsp cinnamon

Filling

8 tbsp butter

1/3 cup sugar

1 tbsp cinnamon

Directions:

Blend ingredients (except butter in a blender.

Let batter rest for 5 min.

Heat butter in a non-stick pan.

Pour batter into the pan.

Cook for two min.

Flip & cook for 1 minute.

Remove & stack on a warm plate.

Mix cinnamon in a bowl until it is combined.

Stir mixture into softened butter till it becomes smooth.

Spread butter mixture on the center of the crepe.

Roll up & sprinkle 1 tsp of the cinnamon mixture.

Nutrition Info: Calories: 434 kcal Fat: 42 g Protein: 12 g Carbs: 2 g Fiber:1 g

Cheesy thyme waffles

Preparation time: 10 minutes

Cooking time: 7 minutes

Servings: 2

Ingredients:

Two eggs

1/3 cup parmesan cheese

1 tsp garlic powder

2 tsp thyme

1 cup collard greens

1 tbsp olive oil

Two stalks onion

1/2 cauliflower

1/2 tsp salt

1 cup shredded mozzarella cheese

1 tbsp of sesame seeds

1/2 tsp black pepper

Directions:

Cut cauliflower & slice onions.

Add cauliflower to the blender.

Add onions, thyme & collard greens to the blender & pulse again.

Now add the processed mixture to a bowl.

Mix it well to form a smooth batter.

A heat waffle iron.

Pour the mixture into the waffle iron, ensuring that it is spread properly.

Cook well & serve hot.

Nutrition Info: Calories: 813 kcal Fat: 61.51 g Protein: 0 g Carbs: 36.95 g Fiber: 13.5 g

Baked egg and asparagus with cheese parmesan

Preparation time: 10minutes

Cooking time: 15minutes

Servings: 3

Ingredients:

30 spears asparagus

Six eggs

3 tbsp parmesan cheese

3/4 tsp salt

3 tsp butter

3 tsp olive oil

3/4 tsp black pepper

Directions:

Preheat microwave up to 400 deg.

Take a small pot of water.

Add salt & add asparagus.

Stir it well.

When water boils again, please remove it from the stove.

Drain asparagus & transfer it to a bowl filled with cold water.

Distribute asparagus.

Among three baking dishes, Top center of the baking dish along with one tsp of butter. Season with salt.

Add eggs to the baking dish.

Bake for 10 min.

Remove it from the microwave.

Top each portion with cheese & black pepper.

Return to microwave & bake it for 7 min.

Serve and enjoy.

Nutrition Info: Calories: 286 kcal Fat: 20 g Protein: 16 g Carbs: 1 g Fiber: 0 g

Creamy cold salad

Preparation time: 10 minutes

Cooking time: 1 minute

Servings: 3

Ingredients:

8 oz salad macaroni

1/4 sliced green onion

1/2 cup red pepper

1/2 cup black olives

1 cup broccoli florets

1/2 cup cucumber

Dressing

1/2 cup mayonnaise

2 tsp vinegar

1/2 tsp kosher salt

1/2 tsp black pepper

1/2 tsp sugar

Directions:

Cook pasta.

When noodles are cooked, add broccoli.

Let broccoli boil 40 sec.

Drain everything.

Rinse well

Stir with mayonnaise, salt, pepper, vinegar & sugar in a bowl.

Add cooked pasta & broccoli in a bowl & stir well.

Add cucumber, olives, pepper, & onion.

Stir again.

Cover & refrigerate until the ready dish is ready to serve.

Stir again before serving.

Enjoy the food!

Nutrition Info: Calories: 297 kcal Fat: 16 g Protein: 5 g Carbs: 31 g Fiber: 2 g

Peppy pepper tomato salad

Preparation time: 5 minutes

Cooking time: 10 minutes

Servings: 4

Ingredients:

One small garlic

1/4 cup olive oil

1 tbsp sherry vinegar

1 tsp balsamic vinegar

Salt and pepper

1 pound tomatoes

1.5 pounds red peppers,

1 tbsp basil

One leaf lettuce

Directions:

Dressing: mix sherry vinegar, garlic, olive oil, balsamic vinegar, salt, and black pepper powder according to taste.

Cut roasted peppers strips.

Toss with dressing.

Add 1/2 basil & toss again.

Remove & discard tough outer leaves.

Wash & dry the leaves & tear them to pieces.

Toss with tomatoes & dressing & basil.

Line platter.

Top with peppers.

Serve slightly chilled.

Nutrition Info: Calories: 191 kcal Fat: 14 g Protein: 11 g
Carbs:16 g Fiber: 3 g

Spinach and grilled feta salad

Preparation time: 10 minutes

Cooking time: 20 minutes

Servings: 1

Ingredients:

1/2 tbsp olive oil

1 oz feta cheese

1 cup shredded mozzarella cheese

One pinch of salt

pepper to taste

One clove garlic

Two ciabatta rolls

1/4 lb spinach

Directions:

Mince garlic & add to a pan with olive oil.

Cook at moderate heat for 3 minutes.

Add frozen spinach & turn heat up.

Cook 5 minutes.

Season it lightly with sea salt & black pepper.

Cut rolls in half.

Add shredded mozzarella & half oz. of feta to bottom

Divide cooked spinach.

Then top each sandwich with a pinch of red pepper plus more
mozzarella.

Place top of ciabatta roll on sandwiches & transfer in a non-stick pan

Fill the pot with water for creating weight.

Place pot on the top of sandwiches to press them.

Flip sandwiches carefully.

Place the weighted pot on top & cook.

Serve hot and enjoy.

Nutrition Info: Calories: 360 kcal Fat: 15.5 g Protein: 19.55 g Carbs: 37.5 g Fiber: 3.35 g

Baked cauliflower

Preparation time: 5 minutes

Cooking time: 20 minutes

Servings: 6

Ingredients:

Five cloves garlic

2 tsp thyme leaves

1/4 tsp red pepper

One head cauliflower

1/4 cup olive oil

2 tsp kosher salt

Directions:

Preheat microwave to 450 deg.

Toss the cauliflower along with olive oil, red pepper & garlic on a baking sheet,

sprinkle with salt & thyme.

Toss again.

Roast till it is golden & tender (20 min). Transfer in serving bowl & now serve.

Nutrition Info: Calories: 108 kcal Fat: 8 g Protein: 2 g Carbs: 6 g Fiber: 2 g

Grapy fennel salad

Preparation time: 8 minutes

Cooking time: 2 minutes

Servings: 3

Ingredients:

2 tbsp Parmesan cheese

1 tbsp lemon

1 tbsp parsley

One fennel bulb or meat slicer

1/8 tsp thyme leaves

2 tbsp olive oil

Directions:

Combine all the ingredients & toss them well.

Now serve in a dish & enjoy.

Nutrition Info: Calories: 57 kcal Fat: 6 g Protein:1 g Carbs:1 g
Fiber:1 g

Detox salad

Preparation time: 15 minutes

Cooking time: 0 minute

Servings: 6

Ingredients:

Detox salad

1/3 cup green onions

One avocado

3 cups kale leaves

1 cup cilantro leaves

2 cups broccoli florets

2 cups red cabbage

1 cup matchstick carrots

1/2 cup almonds

Carrot-ginger dressing

One carrot

1/2 tsp sesame oil

1 tbsp honey

1 tbsp miso

1/4 cup rice wine vinegar

2 tbsp avocado oil

1 tbsp ginger

Kosher salt to taste

Black pepper to taste

Directions:

Salad

1.Add all the ingredients to a large bowl.

2.Toss them all together to mix well.

3.Now serve immediately with carrot & ginger dressing.

4.Take a food processor and place all the ingredients in it. Pulse till it is well smoothed.

5.Add salt & black pepper powder to taste.

6.Add all items to the food processor and blend. Season with salt & pepper powder.

7.Add honey if needed.

8.Serve immediately in a sealed container for seven days.

Nutrition Info: Calories: 361 kcal Fat: 26 g Protein: 4 g Carbs: 35 g Fiber:10 g

Peanut sauce with noodle salad

Preparation time: 15 minutes

Cooking time: 15 minutes

Servings: 6

Ingredients:

Three slices ginger

One garlic

1/4 cup peanut butter

1/4 cup orange juice

3 tbsp lime juice

2 tbsp soy sauce

3 tbsp honey

3 tbsp sesame oil

1 tsp cayenne pepper

1/2 tsp salt

Directions:

Boil drain and chill pasta.

Blend peanut sauce with the blender till it is smooth.

Now place shredded veggies, cilantro, bell pepper & scallions in a bowl.

Cook pasta. Drain and chill under cold running water.

Blend the peanut sauce ingredients using a blender until smooth.

Add the noodles, which are cooled in a bowl & toss again.

Now pour peanut sauce on the top & toss again to combine.

Adjust salt & chili according to taste.

Serve and enjoy.

Nutrition Info: Calories: 286 kcal Fat: 13 g Protein: 3.8 g Carbs: 39.9 g Fiber: 2.6 g

Balela salad

Preparation time: 10 minutes

Cooking time: 0 minute

Servings: 6

Ingredients:

Two cans chickpeas

One can of black beans

Two firm tomatoes

1/2 red onion

1/2 English cucumber

Three cloves garlic

2 tbsp mint

1/4 cup parsley

1 tsp sumac

Salt to taste

Cracked pepper

3 tbsp olive oil

juice of one lemon

pita bread

Hummus

Arugula

Directions:

Mix the chickpeas, onion, tomatoes, mint parsley, and black beans in a bowl.

Add drizzle, olive oil, salt & pepper. Mix them well.

Serve at room temperature. Store in an airtight refrigerator for five days.

We can add a salad with pita bread for extra taste.

Nutrition Info: Calories: 281kcal Fat: 10.3g Protein: 12.6g Carbs: 38.1g Fiber: 12.4g

Blue cheese and arugula salad

Preparation time: 10 minutes

Cooking time: 10 minutes

Servings: 2

Ingredients:

1/4 cup walnuts

1/4 cup blue cheese (crumbled)

1/4 cup cranberries

4 cups arugula

Dressing

1 tbsp red wine vinegar

1 tbsp sherry wine vinegar

1 tsp Dijon mustard

3 tbsp extra virgin olive oil

Directions:

Place all ingredients for dressing in bowl & mix.

Put the arugula in the bowl & pour it into the bowl.

Now toss gently.

Divide into different plates & top it with the remaining ingredients.

Season with salt and pepper. Serve immediately & enjoy.

Nutrition Info: Calories: 415 kcal Fat: 36.1 g Protein: 7 g Carbs: 20.2 g Fiber: 2.7 g

Fennel and seared scallop's salad

Preparation time: 30 minutes

Cooking time: 10 minutes

Servings: 4

Ingredients:

One grapefruit

1 tbsp olive oil

1 tsp raw honey

1/2 tsp chopped fennel seeds

1/4 tsp sea salt

Pinch of black pepper

12 sea scallops

1/2 sliced

4 cups torn red leaf lettuce

12 toasted almonds

Directions:

Strain the grapefruit juice in a cup

For the dressing: Transfer juice into a small bowl & whisk oil, add water, honey, fennel, salt & black pepper.

Set it aside.

Season scallops with remaining fennel & remaining salt.

Heat skillet & brush with remaining oil. Cook scallops for five minutes, flipping halfway, till they become lightly from both sides. Transfer it to a plate & cover it.

Repeat the same with remaining.

Set aside the dressing. In a bowl, toss the fennel & lettuce with the remaining dressing. Divide the fennel salad among the serving plates. Top each salad with the grapefruit pieces & cooked scallops.

Drizzle the reserved dressing over scallops & top with the almonds.

Nutrition Info: Calories: 175 kcal Fat: 6 g Protein: 16 g Carbs: 15 g Fiber: 3 g

Garden salad with orange and olive

Preparation time: 15 minutes

Cooking time: 0 minute

Servings: 4

Ingredients:

Five oranges

4 cups rocket spinach

150 g feta

1 cup olives

2 tbsp olive oil

A pinch of salt

One clove garlic

Directions:

Peel & dice 4 of the oranges

Combine oranges, olives & leaves in a bowl.

Crumble feta over the top of the salad.

Whisk together the final orange juice, olive oil, salt, and as much garlic as you like. Taste & adjust seasoning according to requirement.

Pour dressing on the salad & toss gently to mix well.

Nutrition Info: Calories: 244 kcal Fat: 15 g Protein: 7 g Carbs: 21 g Fiber: 3 g

Ginger yogurt dresses the citrus salad

Preparation time: 15 minutes

Cooking time: 0 minute

Servings: 6

Ingredients:

One grapefruit

Two tangerines

2/3 cup ginger

1/4 cup sugar

2 tbsp honey

Three navel oranges

1/2 cup cranberries

1/4 tsp cinnamon

17.6 oz Greek yogurt

Directions:

Break the grapefruit.

Cut grapefruit threads, cut the tangerine sections into half.

Transfer the grapefruit, all juices & tangerines into a deep serving bowl.

Use a small sharp knife,

Slice oranges into round shapes and slices into quarters.

Add oranges & all juices into a bowl. Mix in cranberries, cinnamon & honey.

Cover & refrigerate for 1 hour.

Then Mix yogurt & ginger in a bowl.

Sprinkle brown sugar & cranberries.

Nutrition Info: Calories: 287 kcal Fat: 4 g Protein: 7 g Carbs: 60 g Fiber: 3 g

Grilled halloumi cheese salad

Preparation time: 10 minutes

Cooking time: 5 minutes

Servings: 4

Ingredients:

Salad

8 oz Halloumi cheese

1 cup black olives

1/2 cup green olives

2 cups tomatoes

4 cups arugula

1 tbsp olive oil

4 cups shishito peppers

1 cup mint leaves

1/2 cup chives

Honey Citrus Dressing

One garlic cloves

1 tsp Dijon mustard

2 tsp honey

2 tsp lemon juice

1/4 cup olive oil

salt and pepper

1 tsp thyme optional

Chili optional

Directions:

Cut down the cheese into 0.5-inch slices and soak them in water if required.

Heat the grill pan & then adds olive oil to it.

Take the cheese slices and grill every slice for 1 to 2 minutes, from one side. Remove the cheese, add the peppers, & increase the temp.

Let the peppers cook for three minutes per side.

Let the peppers cool down & then chop them with the cheese into small cubes.

Mix these with the remaining salad items.

Transfer everything in a small bowl and Enjoy

Nutrition Info: Calories: 463 kcal Fat: 36 g Protein: 12 g Carbs: 27 g Fiber: 12 g

www.ingramcontent.com/pod-product-compliance
Lightning Source LLC
Chambersburg PA
CBHW050756030426
42336CB00012B/1844